BURN SURGERY NUTRITION

Comprehensive Guide Unlocking The Secrets of nutrition after Surgery Success, Nourishing Meal Plans, Recipes And Practical Tips For Optimal Health And Wellness)

DR. ALLAN FREDA

Contents

A Comprehensive Guide to Optimal Post-Surgery Diet for Newly Diagnosed" offers priceless insights into creating a healing-focused diet, especially for people recovering from burn surgery.

It explores the role that nutrition plays in the healing process, providing professional guidance, meal plans, and therapeutic recipes to maximize post-surgery wellness.

The book covers both short-term and long-term nutritional needs to support continued recovery and general health.

Disclaimer

The information in this book is for informational purposes only and should not replace professional medical advice, diagnosis, or treatment. Always consult your physician or a qualified health provider regarding any medical concerns. Do not disregard professional medical advice or delay seeking it based on information in this book.

The author does not endorse or have affiliations with any mentioned entities. References are for informational purposes only.

Consult your healthcare provider before making dietary or lifestyle changes, especially during recovery from surgery, as individual needs vary.

Results may vary, and the information provided is not guaranteed to produce specific outcomes.

By reading this book, you acknowledge and agree to consult your healthcare provider before implementing any information herein.

For further guidance, consult your healthcare provider or reputable medical websites for reliable information on surgery recovery diets.

CHAPTER 1
BURN SURGERY NUTRITION - AN INTRODUCTION

A vital component of the all-encompassing care given to patients receiving burn surgery is nutrition; appropriate nutrition is essential for promoting the healing process, boosting immunity, and lowering the likelihood of complications. In this extensive manual, we will examine the significance of nutrition in burn recovery, investigate how burn injuries affect nutritional status, and comprehend how particular dietary approaches can promote healing and long-term wellness for burn victims.

Recognizing the Significance of Diet in Burn Healing

Adequate nutrition supports cellular repair, tissue regeneration, and immune function—all essential components of burn wound healing—and is fundamental to the healing process, especially in cases of severe burns where the body's metabolic demands are significantly increased. In the absence of adequate nutrition, the body may find it difficult to handle the extensive physiological stress imposed by burn injuries, which could result in delayed wound healing, increased susceptibility to infections, and compromised overall health.

Optimizing nutrition is crucial in reducing the metabolic effects of burn injuries and promoting favorable outcomes in terms of wound healing and recovery.

Burn injuries cause a cascade of metabolic changes that include hypermetabolism, increased breakdown of proteins, and altered utilization of nutrients. The body's energy requirements increase in response to the injury, requiring a higher caloric intake to fuel the healing process. Additionally, burns disrupt the body's ability to retain essential nutrients and maintain fluid balance, further exacerbating the risk of malnutrition and dehydration.

An Overview of Burn Injuries and How They Affect Diet

Burn injuries are defined as skin and subcutaneous tissue damage resulting from exposure to heat, chemicals, electricity, or radiation. The degree of physiological and metabolic disruptions that patients experience can vary greatly, and this can have a significant effect on their nutritional status. Factors such as tissue damage, depth of burn, and the existence of accompanying injuries can all affect the degree of metabolic disturbances and nutritional needs.

Burn injuries cause the skin to become damaged, which compromises the skin's ability to act as a barrier against infection and fluid loss. Severe burns also cause increased oxidative stress, the release of pro-inflammatory cytokines, and metabolic dysregulation. These physiological changes lead to a state of hypermetabolism, where the body uses more energy than usual, resulting in rapid weight loss, muscle wasting, and depletion of essential nutrients.

To support the healing process after burn injuries, nutrition plays a multifaceted role. Enough macronutrient, micronutrient, and fluid intake is necessary to promote tissue repair, modulate inflammation, and enhance immune function. Protein is especially important for wound healing and tissue regeneration because it provides the building blocks needed for collagen synthesis and cellular repair. Carbohydrates are the main energy source, powering metabolic processes and maintaining lean body mass during times of increased catabolism. Healthy fats provide essential fatty acids that support cellular membrane integrity and modulate inflammation, which contributes to the best healing results.

Apart from macronutrients, micronutrients like vitamins and minerals are also important for wound healing and immune function. For instance, zinc plays a role in immune regulation and cellular proliferation, while vitamin C is necessary for collagen synthesis and antioxidant defense.

Adequate consumption of vitamins A and E is also important for skin integrity and preventing oxidative damage. Micronutrients like selenium, copper, and iron are important for enzymatic reactions and antioxidant defense mechanisms, which are crucial for preventing the oxidative stress brought on by burn injuries.

In addition to macronutrients and micronutrients, hydration status is an important factor to take into account when managing patients undergoing burn surgery and optimizing their nutritional support.

Sufficient fluid intake is necessary to maintain blood volume, facilitate nutrient transport, and support tissue perfusion. Inadequate hydration can hinder wound healing, raise the risk of complications like renal failure and electrolyte imbalances, and negatively impact overall patient outcomes.

nutrition is critical to the management of burn injuries because it affects the body's reaction to trauma, wound healing, and overall recovery. Healthcare professionals can help patients successfully navigate the challenges of burn recovery by offering tailored nutrition support, incorporating healing recipes and meal plans, and leveraging expert insights.

It is crucial to understand how burn injuries affect nutritional status and to put appropriate dietary strategies into practice to optimize outcomes and promote long-term wellness in patients undergoing burn surgery.

CHAPTER 2
ASSESSING NUTRITIONAL NEEDS IN PATIENTS WITH BURNS

Since burn patients' bodies need extra nutrients to repair damaged tissue and fight infection, nutrition is important to their recovery. To give burn patients the best care and support possible, nutritional needs must be assessed using a variety of techniques and instruments, determining precise macronutrient and micronutrient requirements, and taking into account variables that may have an impact on these needs.

Nutritional Evaluation Techniques and Resources:

The evaluation of burn patients' nutritional status necessitates a thorough methodology that incorporates both objective and subjective measurements. One of the subjective approaches is the use of dietary history interviews, in which medical practitioners learn about the patient's usual food intake, preferences, and any difficulties they may have in eating. These interviews are useful in detecting any malnourishment or deficiencies that may have existed before the patient's recovery.

Biochemical tests, such as blood tests for protein levels, electrolytes, and micronutrient concentrations, offer insights into the patient's metabolic status and nutrient deficiencies.

Clinical evaluations assess physical signs of malnutrition, such as muscle wasting, edema, and impaired wound healing, to further guide nutritional interventions. Anthropometric measurements, such as height, weight, and body composition analysis, provide valuable data on the patient's nutritional status and help track changes over time.

Determining the Needs for Macronutrients and Micronutrients:

The body's metabolic demands are greatly increased by burn injuries, resulting in hypermetabolism and the catabolism of lean body mass. Consequently, burn patients need higher levels of macronutrients to support energy production, tissue repair, and immune function.

Carbohydrates are the main fuel source, providing energy for cellular activities and preventing protein breakdown; adequate intake of proteins is important for wound healing, muscle regeneration, and immune response; and fats are concentrated energy and help absorb fat-soluble vitamins, which are important for immune function and tissue repair.

Micronutrients like vitamins A, C, and E, zinc, and selenium play important roles in immune function, antioxidant defense, and collagen synthesis, all of which are essential for wound healing. Deficiencies in these micronutrients can impair the healing process and increase the risk of complications in burn patients.

Therefore, assessing micronutrient status and providing supplementation when necessary are essential components of nutritional management in burn care. Burn patients also require adequate intake of macronutrients in addition to micronutrients to support various metabolic processes and maintain overall health.

Pre-existing medical conditions, such as diabetes, renal insufficiency, or cardiovascular disease, can impact nutrient metabolism and require specialized dietary interventions to manage. Burn patients may have unique nutritional needs due to their increased risk of malnutrition and impaired immune function.

The severity and extent of the burn injury, the patient's age, and the presence of comorbidities can all have an impact on the nutritional needs of burn patients. Severe burns covering a large body surface area result in higher metabolic rates and increased nutrient losses through wound exudate, leading to greater nutritional requirements.

Additionally, the presence of comorbidities like infections, organ dysfunction, or systemic inflammatory response syndrome (SIRS) can exacerbate the metabolic stress on burn patients and increase their nutritional needs.

SIRS can cause systemic inflammation and metabolic derangements, requiring adjustments in nutritional support to mitigate these effects. Infections increase energy expenditure and nutrient requirements. Organ dysfunction may impair nutrient absorption and utilization.

Healthcare professionals can create customized nutrition plans to support optimal recovery and long-term wellness by using appropriate assessment methods and understanding the unique macronutrient and micronutrient needs of burn patients. In general, assessing the nutritional needs of burn patients requires a multidisciplinary approach that takes into account various factors influencing metabolism, nutrient requirements, and healing processes.

CHAPTER 3
DIETARY APPROACHES FOR BURN HEALING

Nutrition is critical to the healing process for burn patients. After a burn injury, the body requires more nutrients because of the increased metabolic demands for immune system function and tissue repair. Poor nutrition can delay wound healing, make a patient more vulnerable to infections, and lengthen the recovery period. For this reason, creating a customized post-surgery diet plan is crucial to maximizing recovery and fostering long-term wellness.

Creating a Menu for the Best Nutrition:

Planning a menu is a critical part of making sure burn patients receive the nutrition they need for a full recovery. To meet the increased energy and nutrient requirements, a well-balanced diet should include a variety of nutrient-rich foods from all food groups.

Whole foods, such as fruits, vegetables, whole grains, lean proteins, and healthy fats, are important sources of the vitamins, minerals, and antioxidants needed for healing and immune function. Including a diverse range of foods also helps prevent nutrient deficiencies and supports general health.

Incorporating culturally appropriate foods can improve dietary adherence and satisfaction, leading to better outcomes in the recovery process.

When meal planning for burn patients, it is important to take into account their specific dietary preferences, allergies, and dietary restrictions.

Working with a registered dietitian can help create customized meal plans that meet the patient's nutritional needs while accommodating any particular dietary concerns.

Since burn injuries frequently result in increased energy expenditure and protein losses, it is important to meet protein needs by including high-calorie, high-protein foods in the diet to support wound healing and tissue repair.

Protein is especially important for immune system stimulation, collagen synthesis, and the rebuilding of damaged tissues, so it is important to include foods high in protein in every meal and snack, such as lean meats, poultry, fish, eggs, dairy products, legumes, nuts, and seeds.

Apart from protein, adding high-calorie foods can help burn patients meet their increased energy needs, particularly those who have sustained extensive injuries or are undergoing surgery. Nut butter, avocados, seeds, avocado oil, coconut oil, and fatty fish are healthy sources of calories.

You can increase the number of calories in meals and snacks by adding calorie-dense items like avocado slices to sandwiches, drizzling olive oil over salads, or blending nut butter into smoothies.

Ingredients Packed with Nutrients for Quick Healing:

Nutrient-dense foods are rich in vitamins, minerals, antioxidants, and phytochemicals that play important roles in immune function, tissue repair, and inflammation modulation; including a variety of colorful fruits and vegetables, whole grains, lean proteins, and healthy fats can help ensure burn patients receive a wide array of essential nutrients to support optimal recovery. Including nutrient-dense ingredients in the diet is essential for promoting accelerated healing and supporting overall health during the recovery process.

Nutrient-dense foods that are very helpful for burn rehabilitation include the following:

• Rich in antioxidants, vitamin K, and vitamin C, dark leafy greens like spinach, kale, and Swiss chard help to enhance collagen production and wound healing.

• Vibrantly colored fruits, such as mangoes, berries, and citrus fruits; these foods are rich in phytochemicals, antioxidants, and vitamin C, which boost the immune system and lower inflammation.

• Whole grains, which include complex carbohydrates, fiber, vitamins, and minerals for longer-lasting energy and better satiety. Examples of these include brown rice, quinoa, and oats.

• Lean proteins that are high in critical amino acids that are needed for immune system function, muscle synthesis, and tissue repair, and turkey, turkey, tofu, and legumes.

• Good fats, which include omega-3 fatty acids and antioxidants that improve skin health, lower inflammation, and improve nutrient absorption, can be found in foods like avocados, nuts, seeds, and olive oil.

Burn patients can optimize their nutritional intake and aid in their healing process by incorporating these nutrient-dense ingredients into their meals and snacks. Experimenting with different recipes and cooking techniques can help nutrient-rich foods taste better and be more palatable, which will make them more enjoyable and satisfying to eat.

creating a thorough post-surgery diet plan that emphasizes menu planning, incorporating high-calorie, high-protein foods, and including nutrient-dense ingredients is crucial for optimizing nutrition and encouraging accelerated healing in burn patients. Working with a registered dietitian can help customize meal plans to meet specific needs and preferences, guaranteeing optimal nutrient intake and long-term wellness. Burn patients can support their recovery process by emphasizing nutrition and incorporating healing recipes, meal plans, and professional advice.

CHAPTER 4
BURN PATIENT MEAL PREPARATION TECHNIQUES

Meal preparation becomes a crucial part of the recovery process for burn patients when their nutritional needs are met. Well-prepared meals not only guarantee that vital nutrients are ingested but also promote healing and general health. In this section, we will discuss several meal preparation strategies designed with burn patients in mind, with an emphasis on preserving nutrients, modifying texture for dysphagia, and making meals more visually appealing to promote consumption.

Techniques for Cooking to Preserve Nutrients:

Caretakers can help burn patients receive the maximum nutritional benefit from their meals by prioritizing cooking methods that minimize nutrient loss. Steaming, microwaving, and gentle simmering are among the techniques that help retain vitamins, minerals, and other essential nutrients. When possible, incorporate raw or lightly cooked ingredients to further enhance nutrient retention. Burn injuries frequently result in altered nutrient requirements and increased metabolic demands, so it is imperative to preserve as many nutrients as possible during meal preparation.

Dysphagia, or difficulty swallowing, is a common consequence of burn injuries and presents significant challenges when it comes to meal preparation. Food processors or blenders can be used to achieve desired textures, which ensures that meals are safe and palatable for burn patients with dysphagia. Depending on the severity of dysphagia, different texture modifications may be required, ranging from pureed or minced foods to thickened liquids. Incorporating soft, easily digestible foods like well-cooked vegetables, lean meats, and smoothies can help alleviate swallowing difficulties while providing essential nutrients. Additionally, utilizing food processors or blenders to achieve desired textures can help burn patients with dysphagia.

Maintaining appetite and interest in food is crucial for burn patients undergoing recovery, as proper nutrition plays a pivotal role in the healing process. Therefore, it's essential to incorporate strategies to make meals appealing and appetizing, despite any dietary restrictions or challenges.

One effective approach is to focus on presentation, utilizing vibrant colors, varied textures, and creative garnishes to enhance the visual appeal of dishes. Additionally, incorporating flavorful herbs, spices, and seasonings can elevate the taste profile of meals, making them more enticing to burn patients. Offering a diverse range of foods and incorporating patient preferences whenever possible also helps to stimulate appetite and promote enjoyment of meals.

Furthermore, involving burn patients in meal planning and preparation can foster a sense of autonomy and engagement, further enhancing their dining experience. By implementing these tips and strategies, caregivers can create meals that are not only nutritious but also enjoyable, thereby supporting the overall well-being and recovery of burn patients.

CHAPTER 5
SPECIAL DIETARY CONSIDERATIONS

Due to the body's higher metabolic demands and weakened immune system, burn injuries pose special nutritional management challenges.

An ideal diet following surgery is essential for wound healing, preventing complications, and accelerating overall recovery. This extensive guide explores the fundamental ideas of nutrition management for patients undergoing burn surgery, emphasizing fluid balance and hydration management, addressing nutritional deficiencies, supplementation tactics, dietary restrictions, and allergy adaptations.

Controlling Hydration and Fluid Balance

Adequate hydration is crucial to maintain tissue perfusion, support wound healing, and prevent complications like hypovolemia and electrolyte imbalances. In the acute phase of burn injury, aggressive fluid resuscitation is often necessary to prevent hypovolemic shock and maintain organ perfusion. Intravenous fluids containing electrolytes are administered based on the Parkland formula or similar guidelines to replace lost fluids and maintain adequate urine output.

Fluid balance and hydration are critical components of burn surgery nutrition. Burns disrupt the skin's barrier function, leading to increased fluid loss through evaporation and compromised vascular integrity.

After the acute phase, maintaining optimal hydration becomes critical to support metabolic processes and wound healing. Patients may experience increased insensible losses from wound exudates and elevated body temperature, requiring higher fluid intake than usual. Fluid overload and dehydration can be avoided by regularly monitoring fluid balance through serum electrolyte levels, urine output, and clinical assessment. Individual patient factors, such as age, comorbidities, and burn severity, should all be taken into consideration when adjusting fluid status.

To prevent complications like muscle weakness and arrhythmias, electrolyte balance must be carefully maintained in addition to fluid intake.

Electrolyte levels, including sodium, potassium, chloride, and bicarbonate, should be closely monitored and supplemented as needed to correct imbalances. Depending on the patient's needs and clinical status, intravenous electrolyte solutions or oral rehydration solutions may be used. Close coordination between dietitians, nurses, and physicians is crucial to ensuring optimal fluid and electrolyte management for burn surgery patients throughout the continuum of care.

Resolving Inadequate Nutrient intake and Supplementation

Adequate nutrition is essential to support wound healing, preserve lean body mass, and prevent complications like delayed wound closure and infections; however, burn patients frequently face difficulties meeting their nutritional needs due to factors like reduced appetite, impaired gastrointestinal function, and metabolic derangements. Burn injuries can result in profound metabolic disturbances and nutritional deficiencies due to increased catabolism, hypermetabolism, and altered nutrient utilization.

To address nutritional deficiencies in patients undergoing burn surgery, a thorough evaluation of their nutritional status and requirements is necessary. Energy needs are raised in burn patients because of higher metabolic rates and energy expenditure linked to tissue repair and wound healing; calorie requirements are typically calculated using predictive equations adjusted for patient weight, burn size, and clinical factors. Protein requirements are also raised significantly to support immune function, wound healing, and collagen synthesis; high-protein diets, typically supplying 1.5 to 2.0 grams of protein per kilogram of body weight per day, are advised for burn patients to prevent muscle wasting and encourage tissue regeneration.

Apart from macronutrients, micronutrient deficiencies are also common in burn patients and can hinder the healing process and immune system performance. Crucial vitamins and minerals, such as vitamin C, vitamin A, zinc, and selenium, are important for collagen synthesis, antioxidant defense, and immune modulation. Correcting deficiencies and optimizing nutritional status may require supplementation with micronutrients; however, overdoing it can be toxic and have unfavorable effects. The management of nutritional deficiencies in burn surgery patients should be safe and effective, with customized regimens based on laboratory assessments and clinical judgment.

Modifications for Allergies and Dietary Restrictions

Burn patients may have particular dietary requirements or restrictions based on factors such as allergies, intolerances, cultural preferences, and medical conditions. It is crucial to provide personalized nutrition care that accommodates individual dietary needs while optimizing nutritional intake and supporting recovery.

Dietary restrictions and allergies must be carefully considered in burn surgery nutrition in addition to addressing fluid balance, hydration, and nutritional deficiencies.

During the initial nutritional evaluation, dietary restrictions and allergies should be thoroughly assessed, and appropriate modifications made to the meal plan and feeding regimen; if the patient has a known allergy or intolerance, common allergens like nuts, shellfish, dairy, and gluten should be avoided; alternative sources of nutrients should be identified and incorporated into the diet to ensure adequate intake of essential nutrients while avoiding potential allergens.

A registered dietitian or nutrition specialist can work with patients to create customized meal plans that meet their dietary preferences and nutritional needs. When patients have significant dietary restrictions or preferences, such as vegetarianism or veganism, alternative protein sources should be provided to meet their nutritional needs.

Plant-based protein sources, such as legumes, tofu, tempeh, and quinoa, can be included in the meal plan to ensure adequate protein intake and support wound healing.

A multidisciplinary approach involving collaboration between healthcare providers, dietitians, food service staff, and patients is necessary to manage dietary restrictions and allergies in burn surgery nutrition. Patients need to receive appropriate nutrition care that meets their individual needs and promotes optimal recovery and long-term wellness. Healthcare providers can improve patient outcomes and quality of life by addressing nutritional deficiencies, fluid balance, hydration, and dietary restrictions.

CHAPTER 6)
SUPPORTING LONG-TERM REHABILITATION AND REHABILITATION

As patients move from acute care settings to their homes, it becomes critical to make sure they receive adequate nutrition to support healing, prevent complications, and promote long-term wellness. This involves not only providing essential nutrients but also educating patients on lifestyle modifications and integrating nutrition into their overall burn care plans. Burn injuries can result in significant physiological and metabolic changes that call for a comprehensive approach to nutrition for optimal recovery and rehabilitation.

Making the Switch to Homemade Meals

Transitioning from hospital-based nutrition to home-cooked meals marks a crucial phase in the recovery journey of burn patients.

Home-cooked meals offer the advantage of personalized nutrition tailored to individual needs and preferences, promoting adherence to dietary recommendations while enhancing the overall eating experience. However, this transition requires careful planning and guidance to ensure patients maintain optimal nutritional intake.

Caregivers and healthcare professionals play a pivotal role in educating patients about healthy cooking techniques, ingredient selection, portion control, and meal planning strategies. Emphasizing the importance of incorporating a variety of nutrient-rich foods, such as lean proteins, whole grains, fruits, and vegetables, can help meet the increased energy and nutrient demands associated with burn recovery. Additionally, addressing potential barriers to cooking, such as limited mobility or access to kitchen facilities, is essential in facilitating a smooth transition to home-cooked meals.

Changes in Lifestyle for Long-Term Health and Well-Being

Beyond dietary considerations, supporting long-term recovery and rehabilitation following burn injuries entails implementing lifestyle modifications that promote sustained health and well-being. This encompasses various aspects such as physical activity, stress management, adequate sleep, and smoking cessation.

Encouraging patients to engage in regular physical activity, within the limits of their medical condition, can aid in maintaining muscle mass, improving mobility, and enhancing overall quality of life. Moreover, stress management techniques, such as relaxation exercises or mindfulness practices, can help mitigate the psychological impact of burn injuries and promote emotional well-being. Adequate sleep is also crucial for recovery, as it facilitates tissue repair and regeneration, supports immune function, and enhances cognitive function. Addressing sleep disturbances through sleep hygiene practices or appropriate interventions can optimize recovery outcomes. Additionally, supporting patients in smoking cessation efforts is paramount, as smoking can impair wound healing, increase the risk of complications, and hinder overall rehabilitation progress. By addressing these lifestyle factors holistically, healthcare professionals can empower burn patients to adopt healthier habits that contribute to long-term wellness and resilience.

Including Nutrition in Thorough Burn Care Plans

Integrating nutrition into comprehensive burn care plans involves a multidisciplinary approach that encompasses various healthcare professionals, including dietitians, physicians, nurses, and therapists. Collaborative efforts are essential to address the complex nutritional needs of burn patients throughout the continuum of care, from the acute phase to long-term rehabilitation.

This entails conducting thorough nutritional assessments, developing individualized nutrition care plans, monitoring nutritional status, and providing ongoing education and support.

 In the acute phase, nutrition support may involve enteral or parenteral nutrition to meet increased energy and protein requirements and support wound healing.

 As patients transition to rehabilitation, emphasis is placed on optimizing oral intake, promoting self-management skills, and addressing nutritional deficiencies or malnutrition. Furthermore, integrating nutrition education into burn prevention programs can help raise awareness about the importance of healthy eating habits and lifestyle choices in reducing the risk of burn injuries. By incorporating nutrition into comprehensive burn care plans, healthcare teams can enhance the overall quality of care and promote better outcomes for burn patients.

Ultimately, promoting long-term recovery and rehabilitation for burn patients necessitates a multimodal strategy that takes into account nutritional, lifestyle, and psychosocial factors. Among the crucial elements of this multimodal strategy are the shift to home-cooked meals, lifestyle modifications, and the integration of nutrition into comprehensive burn care plans. Through education, counseling, and support, medical professionals can enable burn patients to make decisions about their diet and way of life that will ultimately promote optimal recovery and long-term wellness.

CHAPTER 7

RECIPES FOR NUTRITION AND HEALING

A thorough understanding of the post-surgery diet is essential when thinking about burn surgery nutrition to ensure the best possible healing and recovery.

Since burn injuries frequently cause significant metabolic stress and increased nutritional needs, a well-designed post-surgery diet is an essential part of the treatment plan and can help promote wound healing, lower the risk of complications, and improve overall well-being.

This comprehensive guide covers a variety of topics related to nutrition after burn surgery, including meal plans, nutrient-dense recipes, and expert advice for long-term wellness.

Smoothies and shakes are great choices for post-burn patients because they are highly digestible and concentrated sources of nutrients.

You can tailor these drinks to your needs by adding fruits, vegetables, protein powders, and healthy fats. Smoothies are a convenient way for people who have trouble chewing or swallowing to get the nutrients they need without feeling uncomfortable. You can also add ingredients like Greek yogurt, nut butter, and avocados to boost the calorie and protein content of smoothies, which will help support the body's increased energy requirements during the healing process. Including fruits and vegetables that are high in antioxidants, like berries and leafy greens, can also help reduce inflammation and s

For those recovering from burn surgery, soups, and stews are not only comforting but also incredibly nutritious options.

Since they are often easy to digest, they are also great for those with reduced appetites or gastrointestinal problems. By incorporating a variety of vegetables, lean proteins, and whole grains, soups, and stews can offer a balanced mix of essential nutrients necessary for healing and recovery. Carrots, celery, onions, and garlic, for example, not only add flavor but also provide vitamins, minerals, and phytonutrients that support immune function and tissue repair. Adding protein sources, like chicken, turkey, or tofu, can help meet increased protein requirements, promoting muscle repair and regeneration. Adding whole grains, like brown rice, quinoa, or barley

Main Courses Packed with Protein and Sides:

Protein is a crucial nutrient for individuals recovering from burn surgery, as it plays a vital role in tissue repair, immune function, and muscle synthesis. Including protein-rich main courses and sides in post-surgery meals is essential for meeting increased protein needs and supporting optimal healing. Lean sources of protein such as poultry, fish, lean beef, eggs, and legumes should be incorporated into meals to provide essential amino acids necessary for tissue regeneration.

Grilled chicken breast, baked fish, or tofu stir-fry are excellent main course options that deliver high-quality protein without excess fat or calories. Pairing protein-rich main courses with nutrient-dense sides such as steamed vegetables, roasted sweet potatoes, or quinoa salad creates a well-balanced meal that promotes healing and satisfies hunger. Incorporating a variety of protein sources and pairing them with complementary sides ensures that individuals recovering from burn surgery receive adequate nutrition to support their recovery process.

Snacks and desserts can play a significant role in providing additional calories, nutrients, and enjoyment for individuals recovering from burn surgery. Choosing nourishing snacks that are high in protein, healthy fats, and complex carbohydrates can help maintain energy levels and prevent muscle wasting during the healing process.

Nutrient-dense options such as Greek yogurt with fruit, mixed nuts, cheese, and whole grain crackers, or hummus with raw vegetables make excellent choices for between-meal snacks. These options provide a balance of macronutrients and micronutrients, supporting overall nutritional needs and promoting satiety.

Additionally, incorporating healthy desserts such as fruit parfaits, chia seed pudding, or dark chocolate-dipped fruit can satisfy cravings for sweets while providing antioxidants and other beneficial nutrients.

Opting for homemade versions of desserts allows for control over ingredients and sugar content, ensuring they align with dietary goals and support optimal healing and recovery.

By including a variety of nourishing snacks and desserts in the post-surgery diet, individuals can enhance their nutritional intake and overall well-being during the recovery process.

a well-balanced diet is crucial for patients recovering from burn surgery to facilitate wound healing, lower the risk of complications, and support long-term wellness.

Rich in nutrients, recipes like smoothies, soups, main courses high in protein, and nourishing snacks and desserts provide an easy and tasty way to meet increased nutritional needs.

These recipes, when combined with a comprehensive post-surgery diet plan, allow patients to maximize their nutritional intake and effectively support their recovery process. Individualized guidance and support in the form of counseling with a registered dietitian or healthcare provider can further help to ensure that nutritional objectives are met and overall health is preserved during the healing process.

CHAPTER 8
HOLISTIC APPROACHES TO BURN RECOVERY: BEYOND THE PLATE

In addition to being physically demanding, burn injuries can also be emotionally and psychologically taxing. The road to recovery is not just about healing physical wounds; it is about using holistic methods that take care of the mind, body, and spirit. This extensive guide explores a variety of non-traditional medical treatment approaches, emphasizing mindful eating, herbal and nutritional supplements, and complementary therapies to promote general wellness during the burn recovery process.

Healing Mindful Eating Techniques

To facilitate healing and promote overall well-being, mindful eating practices can be very helpful to burn survivors.

Mindful eating entails paying full attention to the experience of eating and drinking, both internally and externally. It also encourages people to fully engage their senses, Savoring each bite and appreciating the nourishment it provides. Mindful eating can help burn survivors reestablish a positive relationship with food and promote a sense of control during the recovery process.

In addition, mindful eating highlights the significance of paying attention to the body's signals of hunger and fullness. Burn injuries frequently cause disruptions to regular eating patterns, which can result in changes in appetite and dietary restrictions. By paying attention to these signals, people can better control their food intake and make sure they meet their nutritional needs without going over or under. Mindful eating also promotes awareness of emotional triggers for eating, which can help people distinguish between emotional cravings and physical hunger.

Adding mindfulness to mealtime routines can also improve the overall dining experience for burn survivors. Having a distraction-free, peaceful space can help people relax and reduce stress—a crucial skill during the recovery phase. Gratitude for the food that is being consumed can help foster a positive outlook and accelerate the healing process.

Supplementing with Herbs and Nutrients to Strengthen Recovery

Herbal and nutritional supplements can support burn recovery in addition to a well-balanced diet. Research has demonstrated the anti-inflammatory, antioxidant, and immune-boosting effects of certain vitamins, minerals, and botanicals, which can help with tissue repair and promote overall healing.

While whole foods should be the primary source of protein, supplemental protein powders or shakes may be recommended to ensure sufficient intake, particularly for individuals with increased protein needs due to extensive burns or muscle loss.

Protein is one important nutrient that deserves special attention in burn recovery. Protein is necessary for tissue regeneration and wound healing, making adequate intake crucial for burn survivors.

Another nutrient that has been shown to have significant effects on burn recovery is vitamin C. Packed with antioxidant properties, vitamin C guards against oxidative damage from free radicals, which can worsen inflammation and hinder healing. Furthermore, vitamin C is essential for collagen synthesis, which promotes the growth of new, healthy tissue at the burn injury site.

Aloe vera, for example, has long been used topically to soothe burns and promote skin regeneration; when taken orally, aloe vera may also exert anti-inflammatory effects internally, further supporting the body's healing process.

Several other herbal remedies have also shown promise in supporting burn healing and reducing associated symptoms.

Complementary Medicine to Promote General Health

Apart from diet and supplements, a variety of complementary therapies—which include massage therapy, acupuncture, aromatherapy, yoga, and other modalities—can support overall wellness during burn recovery and supplement conventional medical treatment.

When administered by a trained professional, massage therapy can be customized to meet the specific needs and preferences of burn survivors, offering both physical and emotional benefits.

For example, gentle massage techniques can help prevent scar tissue formation and improve mobility in the surrounding tissues, as well as reduce pain and discomfort associated with burn injuries while promoting relaxation and improving circulation to the affected area.

Another complementary therapy that has gained popularity is acupuncture, which stimulates particular acupoints along the body's meridians to help balance the body's energy flow, thereby reducing stress and pain during burn recovery. Studies have shown that acupuncture may also improve wound healing by boosting blood flow to the affected area and regulating the inflammatory response.

Aromatherapy is the use of plant-based essential oils to support mental, physical, and emotional health. For burn survivors who are experiencing pain, anxiety, or insomnia, oils like lavender and chamomile have calming and anti-inflammatory properties that can help. These oils can be applied topically or inhaled to promote relaxation, lower stress levels, and better-quality sleep, all of which can aid in the body's healing process.

In addition to offering psychological benefits, such as assisting individuals in coping with stress, anxiety, and trauma related to their burn injury, yoga also integrates physical postures, breathing techniques, and meditation to promote overall health and well-being. For burn survivors, gentle yoga practices can help improve flexibility, strength, and range of motion, which may be compromised due to scar tissue formation and immobilization.

Ultimately, burn survivors can optimize their recovery and improve their general well-being by incorporating herbal and nutritional supplements, complementary therapies, and mindful eating practices into their treatment plans.

This comprehensive guide offers a roadmap for navigating the complexities of burn recovery, practical strategies, and expert insights for long-term wellness and healing. burn recovery entails more than just physical healing; it requires a holistic approach that addresses the mind, body, and spirit.

CHAPTER 9
BUILDING A SUPPORTIVE CULINARY ENVIRONMENT

In the context of nutrition following burn surgery, the patient's recuperation and general health depend greatly on the creation of a supportive culinary environment. This environment includes not only the actual kitchen but also the emotional and social support that comes from family, caregivers, and medical professionals. By involving family and caregivers in meal preparation, establishing a healing environment in the kitchen, and offering resources for ongoing education and support, patients can benefit from a more seamless transition to optimal post-surgery nutrition and long-term wellness.

Getting family members and caregivers involved in meal preparation is important for burn surgery patients' recovery because family members are frequently the primary caregivers, offering emotional support, helping with daily tasks, and supporting the patient's rehabilitation process.

In terms of nutrition, family members' meal preparation helps the patient feel less alone and more empowered.

A collaborative approach to meal preparation ensures that the patient receives adequate nutrition while also providing opportunities for shared experiences and family bonding. Simple tasks like chopping vegetables or setting the table can be as simple as encouraging family members to research and prepare nutritious recipes tailored to the patient's dietary needs.

In addition, meal preparation with family members and caregivers offers a way to educate and develop skills.

Family members can better support the patient's dietary needs during the immediate post-surgery phase and throughout the long-term recovery process by learning about the nutritional requirements specific to burn surgery recovery and how to incorporate them into everyday meals.

Creating a Restorative Environment in the Kitchen

The kitchen is the center of the home, and fostering a healing environment in this area is critical to fostering recovery and general well-being, particularly for those undergoing burn surgery.

A healing kitchen is orderly, spotless, and filled with nourishing ingredients that aid in the body's natural healing process.

Frequent cleaning and sanitization of cooking surfaces, utensils, and food storage areas help reduce the risk of contamination and ensure that meals are prepared safely and healthily. Keep your kitchen clean and hygienic to prevent infections, which can pose serious risks to burn surgery patients whose immune systems may be compromised.

A well-organized kitchen not only expedites meal preparation but also encourages mindfulness and intentionality in food choices. By keeping necessary ingredients easily accessible and setting up cooking utensils ergonomically, caregivers can reduce stress and maximize efficiency in meal preparation, freeing them up to concentrate more on providing nourishing meals for the patient. Organization is just as important to creating a healing atmosphere in the kitchen as cleanliness.

Additionally, the body needs nourishing ingredients to support the healing process and to promote overall wellness. The cornerstones of a post-surgery diet should consist of fresh fruits and vegetables, lean proteins, whole grains, and healthy fats. These nutrients offer vital vitamins, minerals, antioxidants, and proteins that support immune system function, tissue repair, and overall recovery.

Ongoing education and support are critical elements in the path to long-term wellness and optimal post-surgery nutrition. Burn surgery patients and their caregivers need to have access to trustworthy resources that offer customized advice on diet, meal planning, and lifestyle modifications.

Nutrition counseling from burn care specialists is a great way to receive ongoing education and support. They can provide individualized advice on dietary strategies to promote healing, manage potential complications like weight loss or malnutrition, and improve long-term health outcomes. Patients and caregivers can also acquire the knowledge and skills needed to make decisions about what to eat and how to prepare meals by working closely with a registered dietitian or nutritionist.

Apart from tailored nutrition counseling, community-based programs and support groups can be an invaluable source of assistance and motivation for burn surgery patients and their families. These groups provide a forum for the exchange of experiences, information, and connections with like-minded individuals.

Through participation in support groups, patients and caregivers can obtain valuable perspectives, useful advice, and emotional support that can help them better manage the intricacies of burn surgery recovery.

Additionally, websites, blogs, and social media platforms can be a great source of information and inspiration for patients recovering from burn surgery and their caregivers.

These platforms can provide a wealth of information and support at the touch of a button, including educational articles, cooking tutorials, recipe ideas, and discussion forums. By utilizing these online resources, patients and caregivers can access a variety of viewpoints and suggestions to help them on their path to long-term wellness and optimal post-surgery nutrition.

creating a supportive culinary environment is crucial to promoting optimal post-surgery nutrition and long-term wellness for patients who have had burn surgery. Patients can receive the emotional support and nutritional support they require to thrive during their recovery process by involving family and caregivers in meal preparation, fostering a healing environment in the kitchen, and providing resources for ongoing education and support. Collaboration, education, and community support can help burn surgery patients and their caregivers work together to optimize nutrition, promote healing, and improve overall quality of life.

CONCLUSION

This thorough guide has shed light on the vital role that nutrition plays in promoting the healing process, highlighting the need for individualized meal planning and nutrient-dense foods.

Every chapter has offered priceless insights and doable solutions for maximizing post-surgery diet, from comprehending the complex effects of burn injuries on nutritional needs to putting specific meal preparation skills into practice and addressing dietary problems.

In addition, the provision of professional advice, meal planning, and therapeutic recipes highlights the holistic approach to rehabilitation, emphasizing the significance of nourishing the mind and soul in addition to the body.

The incorporation of nutrition into comprehensive care regimens is essential as patients move toward long-term recovery and rehabilitation, since it promotes continued health and well-being outside of the parameters of medical intervention.

In the end, we can enable patients to set out on a path toward recovery, resilience, and a revitalized sense of life by cultivating a supportive culinary environment and adopting holistic methods of therapy.